Dedicated to

Sisters in Fitness & Health [SIFH] this Change Your Life Guide is for you but is also dedicated to my mom, she believes in everything I do. Without her love and support I would not have known how to do this. Thank you so much, Mrs. Mary Queen Jackson!

Also to my trainer Paul K. Davis of Speed Weight Training Fitness Center, thank you for always pushing me and never taking a I can't for an answer. You have helped to build courage in me that I will now share with the women of SIFH.

To my SIFH, I can't help you get taller, nor can I help you to get shorter, but I can certainly lead you to the physique of your dreams.

For more information about SIFH and our programs visit us on the SIFH website: www.SIFH-Wellness.com.

- Table of Contents

Change Your Life Challenge
Your Weight Loss Guide to Success

If you are currently only eating one to three times a day and you do not eat enough of the right calories, you have probably conditioned your body to hold on to calories which the body stores as fat. The body stores some of the calories because it does not know when it will be getting fuel again and the stored fuel will be used later for energy. Going down this road results in a slow metabolism and *Minimal or No Weight Loss*.

You **MUST** eat five (5) to six (6) small meals each day, approximately every 2 ½ - 3 hours, preferably every 3 hours. Each meal should consist of approximately 300 calories. By eating small meals five (5) to six (6) times a day, the body recognizes that it is getting food regularly and burns those calories. Because of the frequency that you are eating, and providing that you are eating the right combination and portion of food, your metabolism will work at a faster rate resulting in *Weight Loss*.

Reason that We Need Protein in Our Diet

- It is necessary for the building and repair of body tissue.

- It helps produce enzymes, hormones and other substances the body uses.

- It helps regulate body processes such as water balancing, transporting nutrients and making muscles contract.

- It helps keep the body healthy by resisting diseases that are common to malnourished people.

- It helps prevent one from becoming easily fatigued by producing stamina and energy.

Emerging research has hinted that protein may be able to satisfy hunger better than either fats or carbohydrates.

Problems with Excess Protein

- It will be stored as fat.

- Without exercise, the fat will continue to increase.

- It may also result in osteoporosis and kidney stones.

According to Dr. Benardot, "If you consume enough energy from carbohydrates, then the protein that you consume will be used for all the valuable protein related functions, such as synthesis and maintenance of muscle, synthesis of creatine and the creation of hormones and enzymes."

If you do not consume enough carbohydrates energy, the consumed protein will be burned as fuel rather than used for the critical functions mentioned above. Burning protein as fuel causes increase water loss, which can increase risk of dehydration.

What is Carbohydrates?

Carbohydrates are foods that contain simple sugars or starches.

1. Sugars are called *simple carbohydrates* because it absorbs into the blood much faster, providing for some real quick energy. Simple carbohydrates are usually sweet tasting things like cookies, candy and other sugary foods, including many fruits. They can often come with lots of fat and lack important vitamins that your body needs.

2. Starchy carbohydrates are called *complex carbohydrates*. They take longer to release into the blood, therefore giving you energy more slowly. The complex carbohydrates that your body likes to use as fuel are brown rice, oatmeal, sweet potatoes, bread, cereal and pasta. Also good vegetable choices are sweet potatoes, tomatoes, carrots, cucumbers, romaine lettuce and peppers.

Complex carbohydrates are better than simple carbohydrates, because they usually come with lots of vitamins and minerals that your body needs.

Good Carbohydrates

Good carbohydrates are **UNREFINED** and are found in whole natural food such as whole grains, brown rice, quinoa, legumes and starchy vegetables.

Bad Carbohydrates

Bad Carbohydrates are **REFINED** carbohydrates and are usually found in packaged processed foods such as store bought baked goods, crackers, pasta, white bread and white rice. They are usually made with white flour and contain little or no fiber, because the process of turning grain into white flour strips away its fiber and nutrients.

Reason that We Need Carbohydrates in Our Diet

It gives the cells in our body the energy they need. When you eat food that has carbohydrates in them the body breaks the food down into two different types of fuel, immediate fuel and stored fuel.

For energy that you will use immediately, your body takes those carbohydrates and turns them into *glucose*, which is carried into the blood cells and gives you energy to do the things that you do.

Whenever there is left over glucose/fuel, it is saved and stored in the liver and muscles. This is called glycogen. It turns into fat waiting until it is needed. When exercising for a long period of time your body then turns to its reserve tank for fuel, burning those stored fats that have been in reserve.

Reasons that We Need Fats in Our Diet

It is essential to good health and can help protect us against certain disorders and food allergies. Healthy fats are known as the "Good Fats."

We know natural fats as either Saturated or Unsaturated. *Saturated fats* are primarily from animal fats like butter, cream, beef, etc. These are considered to be solid fats and are not good for us in large quantities over time.

Unsaturated fats are mainly oils from vegetables like flaxseed, including the oils that we get from seeds, nuts, eggs, oily fish and leafy green vegetables. These are all needed as they give us the necessary fatty acids that we get from the groups Omega 3 and Omega 6.

According to experts, many of us have a tendency to eat too many saturated fats, because of the packaged and processed foods that we find on our supermarket shelves. In order to ensure a healthy diet, the experts say that we should limit our total fat intake to 30%, with no more than 10% coming from saturated fats. This means that many of us should cut back on our intake of meats, butter, ice cream and commercial products and increase our intake of fish, flaxseed, eggs, avocado, olive oil and coconut oil.

How Can Water Affect Fat-Loss

Water helps to naturally suppress appetite. Stored fat is metabolized with water. Many studies have proven that high water intake does just the opposite. A good rule of thumb is to drink ½ of your body weight in ounces of water. For example, if you weigh 200lbs, you should drink at least 100 ounces of water per day. Increase by 10 – 15 ounce increments over time.

If you have difficulty drinking plain water try infusing your water with cucumbers or fruit. I **do not** recommend any products that contain artificial sweeteners. I enjoy Wisdom brand liquid stevia drops or water enhancers in my water occasionally.

Daily Balanced Meal Consist of:

Protein 40%, Carbohydrates 30%, Fat 30%; recommended by the American Heart Association.

Sample Daily Meal Plan (App. 1400 -1500 cal.)

This is a go-by; build your own meal plan according to your individual caloric needs.

Meal 1: 5 eggs whites and ½ cup of oatmeal **or** 5 egg whites and 1 cup of veggies.

Meal 2: 4 oz. Chicken or turkey **or** 6 oz. fish and ½ cup veggies **or** 1 medium apple or ½ cup blueberries.

Meal 3: 4 oz. Chicken or turkey **or** 6 oz. fish, 1 cup of veggies and 1-cup brown rice or ½ cup sweet potatoes.

Meal 4: 4 oz. Chicken or turkey **or** 6 oz. fish and ½ cup of veggies.

Meal 5: 4 oz. Chicken or turkey **or** 6 oz. fish and 1 cup of veggies.

Note:

Meal 2 or Meal 4 can be either the food or a plant based protein drink. Daily have approximately 300 calories of good fat. Recommendations are coconut oil, almonds or flaxseed.

If you make substitutions to this meal plan, make sure to check the label for protein, carbohydrates, fat, sugar and sodium content. Everything that looks like a substitution may not be an equal substitution.

Food

Farm Raised Tilapia

Farm raised tilapia; one of the most highly consumed fish in America has low levels of beneficial omega-3 fatty acids and, perhaps worse very high levels of omega 6 fatty acids. Tilapia is lower in several vitamins than some other fish. It has no vitamin C, in contrast to the average 4 percent daily value for vitamin C that a serving of salmon and trout provide. Tilapia is also lower in B vitamins, including folate, thiamin, riboflavin, niacin, B-5, B-6 and B-12. Unlike canned salmon, sardines and oysters, tilapia contains no calcium. In addition I am not a supporter of the practices utilized by the fish farm industry and consequently I do not consume any farm raised or genetically modified fish.

Foods to Avoid

Artificial Sweeteners:

Saccharin can be found as Sweet 'N' Low and Sugar Twin. **Aspartame** is found as Crystal Light, NutraSweet and Equal. **Acesulfame potassium or acesulfame-K** is found as Sweet One, Swiss Sweet and Sunett. **Sucralose** is found as Splenda. Do NOT use artificial sweeteners including foods containing high fructose corn syrup.

Condiments:

Ketchup, hot sauce (sugar and sodium contents are high), high calorie salad dressing, mayonnaise.

Refined Foods:

White rice, white flour, white bread, white sugar, corn syrup, refined honey and refined maple syrup.

Acceptable Foods

Natural Sweeteners:

Blackstrap Molasses, raw honey, Wisdom SweetLeaf Stevia (SIFH website)

Condiments:

Balsamic vinegar, mustard (moderation)

Good Fats/Oils:

Flaxseed oil, olive oil, coconut oil, MCT oil (high quality), Omega 3s, nuts, seeds, avocados

Seasoning:

Any natural no sodium seasoning that you like. You can also use green peppers, red peppers and onions, but in moderation.

Foods to Incorporate Once You Reach Your Goal

Snacks:

Consider having an apple, avocado, banana, blueberries, grapes, raisins, almonds or walnuts. Other foods to consider are Greek yogurt, natural peanut butter, beans, lentils and almond milk. Once you have learned to design your own meal plan, the list of foods to incorporate could be endless.

The Don'ts

1. Complex/Starchy carbohydrates should **not** be eaten after 4:30 pm.

2. Complex/Starchy carbohydrates should **not** be eaten alone, pair them with a protein.

3. Don't eat white rice, white potatoes, white bread, white flour, white sugars, etc.

The Do's

1. Purchase a scale and weigh yourself.

2. Purchase a food scale and weigh your foods.

3. Purchase a measuring tape and measure yourself.

4. Purchase a heart rate monitor for your workouts.

5. Journal your food and workouts.

6. Drink tea and water to help with in between meal hunger.

7. Take photos of yourself so that you will have before photos as a reminder of your accomplishments.

Routine for Meal Planning

- Grocery shop every 2 weeks because it saves time and makes meal preparation run smoother.
- Cook once a week so that your meals are always ready and you can eat on schedule.
- Weigh and pack your food in meal size containers.

Note:

Take your prepared food with you everywhere you go (work, shopping, gym, etc.) Pack enough food for the worst-case scenario.

Digestive Enzyme Supplements

When we cook our food, the enzymes in the food are destroyed and our body has to make them *in order to digest our food*. This puts stress on our system, especially since people eat more processed foods and meals that are higher in calories and fats. Digestive enzyme supplements help your system digest your meals more efficiently and deliver the nutrients from your foods to your body.

Importance of Enzymes

Enzymes are one of the most essential elements in our body and are responsible for construction, synthesizing, carrying, dispensing, delivering and eliminating the many ingredients and chemicals our body uses in its daily business of living. It breaks down the food we eat releasing nutrients for energy production and cell growth and repair.

During the First Week of Starting the Plan

During the first week on the plan you may not feel like you are hungry every 2 to 3 hours, however it is *critical* to the process of speeding up your metabolism that you eat. By the second week on the plan you will find yourself hungry and ready to eat in about 2 ½ hours. This is an indication that your metabolism has been jump-started.

Another critical point is that you must do everything possible not to skip a meal. Here is an example of how important it is not to skip a meal, if you are faced with whether to skip a meal or skip a workout, *skip the workout not the meal*.

Stop Emotional Eating

Do not use food to soothe stressful feelings, alleviate boredom or to reward and comfort ourselves.

1. Make a Commitment: Until you have made a commitment to change your behavior, nothing will change.

2. Practice awareness: Make a habit to document what you eat, including your feelings before and afterward.

3. Manage your stress; Positive ways to reduce stress could be exercising, relaxation, getting support from those that care about you, etc.

4. Be physically active: Make sure that you include some kind of physical activities in your day.

5. Create new comforts: make a list of healthy activities you enjoy and whenever you feel that need, treat yourself to something on your list.

6. Eat mini-meals often: it helps to keep your blood sugar and moods stable.

7. Get rid of temptations: do not food shop when you are hungry or stressed. If you plan to eat out plan ahead.

8. Get enough sleep: when you are tired it is easier to give in to emotional eating. Make sure that you get enough rest.

9. Use healthy distractions: do some kind of activity such as taking a walk, listening to music, reading a book, watching a movie, etc.

10. Practice mindfulness: pay attention to your thoughts when you are eating. Eat and chew your food slowly.

11. Get some support: Controlling emotional eating is easier to accomplish with support from others.

Finally, learning how to stop emotional eating and overeating is a life-changing experience. Just make sure to stay on track and enjoy the journey.

Cardiovascular Training

Can interval training boost your calorie-burning power?

Interval training is a powerful tool for novice exercisers and accomplished athletes alike. Here's how it works.

By Mayo Clinic Staff

"Are you ready to shake up your workout routine? Do you wish you could burn more calories without spending more time at the gym? Consider aerobic interval training. Once the domain of elite athletes, interval training has become a powerful tool for the average exerciser, too."

What is Interval Training?

It's not as complicated as you might think. Interval training is simply alternating bursts of intense activity with intervals of lighter activity.

Take walking; if you are in good shape you might incorporate short bursts of jogging into your regular brisk walks. If you are less fit, you might alternate leisurely walking with periods of faster walking. For example, if you are walking outdoors, you could walk faster between certain mailboxes, trees or other landmarks.

What can Interval Training do for me?

Whether you are a novice exerciser or you have been exercising for years, interval training can help you. Here are the benefits:

- **You will burn more calories**. The more vigorously you exercise the more calories you will burn – even if you increase intensity for just a few minutes at a time.
- **You will improve your aerobic capacity.** As your cardiovascular fitness improves, you will be able to exercise longer or with more intensity. Imagine finishing your 60-minute walk in 45 minutes or the additional calories you will burn by keeping up the pace for the full 60 minutes.

- **You will keep boredom at bay.** Turning up your intensity in short intervals can add variety to your exercise routine.
- **You do not need special equipment.** You can simply modify your current routine.

Are the Principles or Interval Training the Same for Everyone?

Yes, but you can take interval training to many levels. If you simply want to vary your exercise routine, you can determine the length and speed of each high-intensity interval based on how you feel that day. After warming up, you might increase the intensity for 30 seconds and then resume your normal pace, for how often and for how long is up to you.

Does Interval Training have Risks?

Interval training is not appropriate for everyone. If you have a chronic health condition or have not been exercising regularly, consult your doctor before trying any type of interval training.

Also, keep the risk of overuse injury in mind. If you rush into a strenuous workout before your body is ready, you may hurt your muscles, tendons or bones. Instead, start slowly. Try just one or two higher intensity intervals during each workout at first. If you think that you are overdoing it, slow down as your stamina improves, challenge yourself to vary the pace. You may be surprised by the results.

The Importance of Strength Training

By Articlesbase

We hear a lot about the importance of exercise for better health. We understand that aerobic exercise is beneficial for heart health and helps to burn fat. But what about adding strength training? How important is it to our overall fitness program?

Many people still have the notion that strength training will make you build big, bulging muscles like you see in bodybuilders. Most people, especially women, do not want to have this look. As a result they stay away from weights.

Nothing could be further from the truth. Strength training helps us to look lean and healthy. Where good nutrition and aerobics help to burn off the fat, strength training helps to tone the muscles that were underneath the fat. You cannot have a toned body without using weight resistance.

Strengthening your muscles does more than just make you look good. It helps you have better posture and strengthens your entire framework. Having strong muscles allows you to carry your body's weight more effectively. Resistance training is a great way to build the muscle your body requires.

Another reason for strength training is to help prevent muscle loss. As we get older we start to lose muscle. And since the muscle helps to support our skeletal system, losing muscle can affect our bones as well. If you plan to live to a ripe old age, it is important to keep your muscles strong so that you are able to have strong bones as well.

However, the natural loss of muscle can be prevented. By using resistance to work your muscles you can help to reverse the muscle lost to aging. You can regain the body you had in your youth by working your muscles as well as practicing good nutrition and aerobic exercise.

Not only will strength training help to build good core muscles, it will help strengthen your bones and increase your metabolism. In fact, strength training will actually help boost your weight loss firing up your fat burning furnace. Studies show that fat burning continues long after you are finished strength training. It also can increase bone density and may help prevent osteoporosis.

As far as those who think that you will look like a bodybuilder if you use weights, there is nothing farther from the truth. Being a bodybuilder is far more complicated than that, it takes specific training and know how. Just lifting weights and no specific training will not make you look like a bodybuilder.

No matter what your fitness goals are, adding resistance training to your routine can help you reach them. You will look better, feel better and have better health by following good nutrition and an exercise program that includes aerobics and strength training.

Note: Consult with your physician before you begin this challenge. Also do more research on your own. You can never have too much knowledge.

Disclaimer

Information contained or provided by this publication is provided on an "as is basis". That means that the information contained on or provided is intended for general consumer understanding and education.   All access to this material is voluntary and at the sole risk of the user.

It is advised that the user seek the advice of a physician or other qualified health care provider with any questions regarding personal health or medical conditions. Never disregard, avoid or delay in obtaining medical advice from your doctor or other qualified health care provider because of something you have read in this publication. If you have or suspect that you have a medical problem or condition, please contact a qualified health care professional immediately.

<u>Thinking</u>

If you think you are beaten, you are;

If you think you dare not, you don't

If you'd like to win, but you think you can't

It's almost a cinch you won't.

If you think you'll lose, you've lost,

For out of the world we find

Success begins with a fellow's will;

It's all in the state of mind.

If you think you are outclassed, you are:

You've got to think high to rise,

You've got to be sure of yourself before

You can ever win a prize.

Life's battles don't always go

To the stronger or faster man,

But soon or later the man who wins

Is the one WHO THINKS HE CAN!

-Walter D. Wintle- 1905

<u>Don't Quit!</u>

When things go wrong, as they sometimes will,

When the road you're trudging seems all uphill,

When the funds are low, and the debts are high,

And you want to smile, but you have to sigh,

When care is pressing you down a bit,

Rest if you must, but don't you quit.

Life is queer with its twist and turns,

As everyone of us sometimes learns,

And many a failure turns about,

When he might have won had he stuck it out;

Don't give up though the pace seems slow,

You may succeed with another blow.

Success is failure turned inside out,

The silver tint of the clouds of doubt,

And you never can tell how close you are,

It may be near when it seems so far;

So stick to the fight when you're hardest hit,

It's when things seem worst, that

You Must Not Quit.

Anonymous

SIS†ERS
IN FITNESS AND HEALTH

SIFH ONLINE CATALOG

Catalog Merchandise can be purchased at *www.SIFH-Wellness.com*

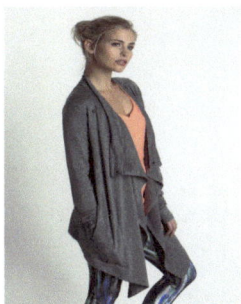

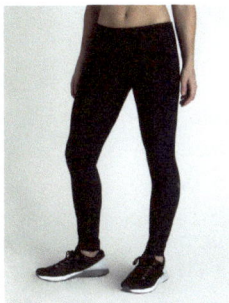

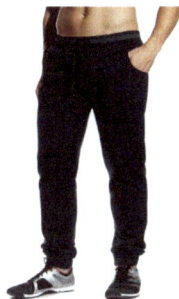

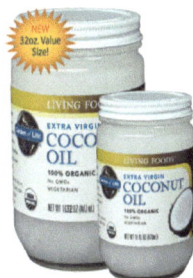

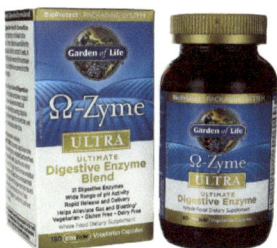

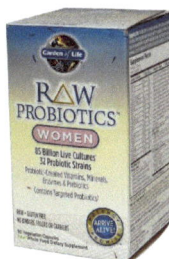

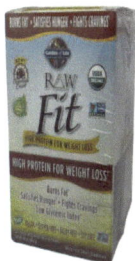

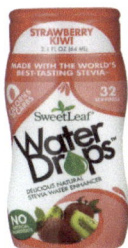

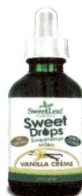